BE YOUR BEST HEALTH ADVOCATE

A JOURNAL EMPOWERING PATIENTS TO SURVIVE HEALTHCARE ANOTHER DAY

Riya Aarini

Disclaimer

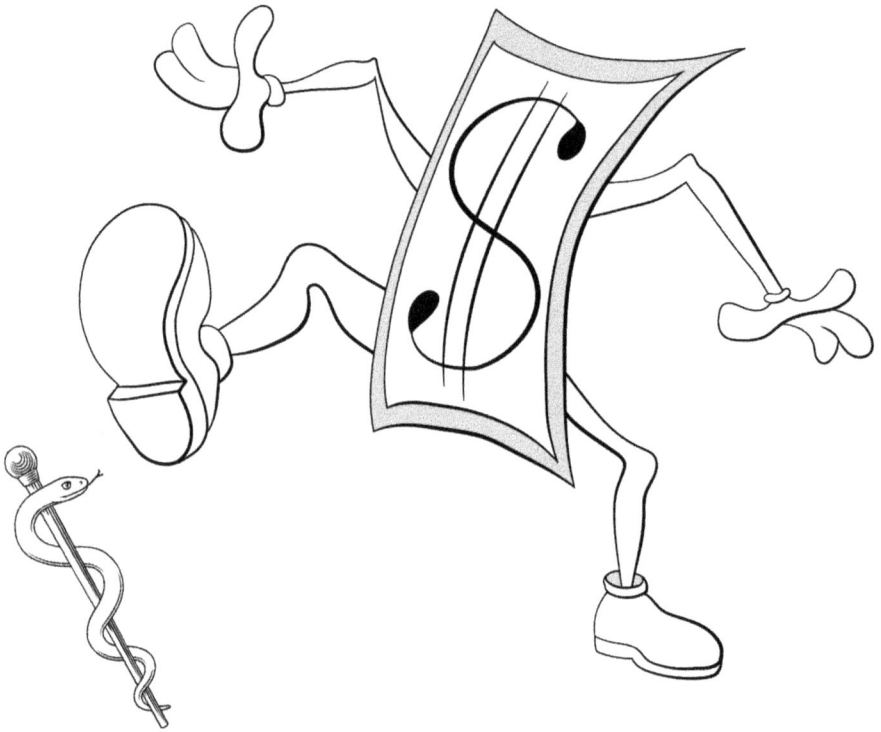

HEALTHCARE IN THE US

Contents

One medicine vital for patients dealing with the medical establishment is a healthy dose of skepticism.

Introduction

Once a patient gave her then-doctor a mug inscribed with, "Please don't confuse your Google search with my medical degree." He laughed and showed it off to his staff. Unbeknownst to her at the time, that doctor had misdiagnosed her for years. Ironically, only after performing extensive online research did she learn he'd been treating her for a condition she never had. He'd extolled the virtues of a medication as if it were manna from heaven—for a disease he wrongly claimed she suffered—never warning her of its subtle yet gradually crushing side effects. As a naive, trusting patient, she failed to realize the medicine she was told she needed for health actually sent it coasting down a jagged ravine like a tumbleweed on its way into the unforgiving chasm of doom. At a pivotal crossroads, she carefully assessed her own well-being, quit the unnecessary treatment, fired the negligent doctor, and is now living her happiest, healthiest life.

But her quality of life had been reduced to that of an unsuspecting housefly caught in the teeth of a Venus flytrap luring it with false promises of blooming health. That Venus flytrap was none other than a torturous healthcare trap that had ensnared her for years, causing her slow, painful demise.

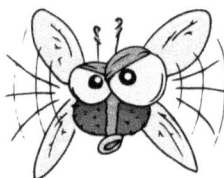

Perhaps if she'd utilized a pro-patient journal like this, she'd have skirted the medical *mistreatment*—well-disguised as medical treatment—sooner.

Today's patients have an abundance of credible health resources at their disposal to help them make informed decisions and avoid sticky snares. By no means are resources always accurate or inaccurate, just as healthcare providers aren't consistently right or wrong. But responsible use of authoritative online resources is among the many tools patients utilize to navigate the complex road of health. They might not allow patients to correctly self-diagnose, but they can increase self-awareness—sometimes helping them learn whether what they experience is due to a genuine medical condition or external factors with no biological basis.

The wealth of consumer-friendly information serves to support patients, who shouldn't feel compelled to accept a medical diagnosis that seems "off" or take medications that do more harm than good.

This journal is not a source of medical advice. It if were, it'd be followed by a $300 charge for fifteen minutes' worth of pages read, a battery of pointless health tests, and might not be in-network with insurance...plus a sneer for good measure.

The advice that doctors never give (but should include in their medical agenda) is that laughter is the best medicine. It's helped humanity cope for eons. No prescription required.

Rather this journal is intended to accompany patients on their health journey, like a cohort rooting them through a tricky phase of life, where a wrong turn can end them up in a horrible sterile environment with whitewashed walls and strange people—wearing masks, gloves, and clogs—who poke and prod at them.

MASKED PERSON 1: "WHAT DO YOU THINK IT IS?"
MASKED PERSON 2: "I DON'T KNOW."
MASKED PERSON 1: "POKE AT IT AGAIN."

This journal helps patients tap into their natural intuitions and organize external resources that give them greater clarity and depth of knowledge about health diagnoses, symptoms, side effects, and treatment options that a sole healthcare resource is unable, unwilling, or has little time to provide. Answering the questions candidly allows patients to hold open conversations with themselves and a reliable medical specialist—from a place of self-awareness, knowledge, and self-empowerment.

People strive to lead their healthiest lives, and most pay dearly for the promise of health—one of the well-worn keys to quality of life. Complete the relevant sections in this guided journal for your own self-fulfillment and to mark progress on your health journey. Or share the content with a trusted healthcare professional. Upon reflection, your answers might just be eye-opening for both you and your provider and create a richer, more satisfying healthcare experience.

Here's to surviving the healthcare industry another day!

1

The Unhealthy Perception of US Healthcare

Healthcare practitioners are like mechanics: some good, others iffy. The good ones diagnose an issue with accuracy and provide an ethical fix. The questionable ones perform unnecessary tests, prescribe excessive treatments, and leave you in worse shape than before. The good and the bad exist in every field—medicine is no exception. That's why it behooves patients to be self-aware of their symptoms and conditions, if any, and advocate for themselves in the best way possible. Of course, it's always a stroke of luck to find a trustworthy professional—whether it's an honest mechanic or a capable healthcare practitioner. But good things in life are as uncommon as sneezing with your eyes wide open.

Contrary to popular opinion, doctors are not oracles that see into the depths of sickness and pull cures out of thin air. They err. They're human. They are swamped with never-ending car payments, are enthusiastic about funding Caribbean vacations, and shop for groceries. Although they might drive fancier vehicles, fly to more exotic destinations, and opt for organic. Still, they are subject to the woes of the human condition—which means *mistakes*...and apathy, greed, ignorance, carelessness....

This is why it's vital patients be proactive about their health. Ask questions, challenge medical experts when doubts arise, and know your patient and human rights. If you struggle to stand up to healthcare professionals, your well-thought-out answers in this journal are starting points of mean muscle, giving you a foundation of self-empowerment and self-awareness to advocate for yourself and your health.

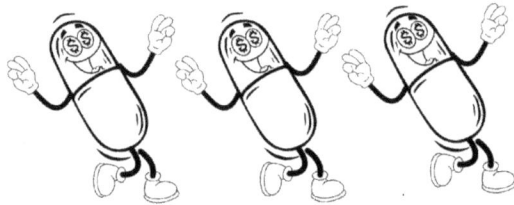

The US respects doctors to such a high degree that a person who merely mentions, "I am a doctor," garners instant reverence from his audience. Eyes sparkle, ears perk up, and body language shifts to give full attention to the healthcare superhero with miraculous healing powers.

The esteem bestowed upon physicians in the US is so high that even dentists, chiropractors, and optometrists sponge off this impressive reputation. A dentist, for instance, introduces herself as, "I am *Dr.* Molly," with such glowing pride—as if emphasizing the word "doctor" elevates her humble status as dentist to all-powerful doctor. Or the chiropractor refers to himself as *Dr. Ken* with the stance of a champ, and the optometrist exhibits a visible whoosh of joy upon being called *Dr. Mirjana*.

Although physicians undergo a few more years of additional training than dentists, chiropractors, and optometrists, it doesn't transform them into miracle workers who cure patients' ills and instantly give them an amazing quality of life. Some doctors *are* helpful and relieve aches and pains with a great deal of skill. As in all professions, however, there are the good, the bad, and the ones that make you scratch your head...quite vigorously.

Americans swoon. "Oh, doctors are the smartest people I know."

Um, really? Some highly trained health specialists fail to distinguish between an inherent medical condition and temporary symptoms caused by external factors—like stress, which can be resolved without creating a needless, lifelong dependency on the broken US healthcare system. Yet they treat the two just the same, destroying the patient's quality of life with rounds of ruthless, unnecessary treatments.

Instead, given the prevalence of misdiagnoses that upend patients' lives for years, gross failures to monitor for harmful side effects, rampant medical abuses, and justified medical malpractice claims, we should take a cautious step back and say, "Oh, you're a *doctor*?"

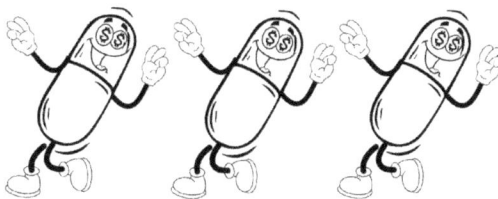

Being a doctor is just a job, like flipping burgers. How often do you see a fast-food worker pay critical attention to the patties sizzling on the grill, ensuring each one glistens with beads of cholesterol-laden grease before gently setting it in the perfect center of a soft, white bun with utmost care? It's rare! Similarly, patients are hard-pressed to find a doctor who applies a high degree of meticulousness to the well-being of every patient. Healthcare workers do enough to keep the lights on, pay their bills, and maintain the prestige that drove them into the field in the first place. This is why patients would be wise to avoid a chancy undercooked burger—and an equally risky subpar doctor.

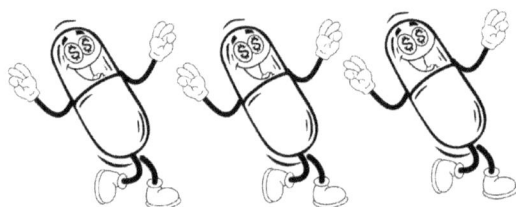

Giving unquestionable authority to a doctor is a grave error—that can lead to the grave! A doctor is trained to detect illness, sometimes even in the absence of illness, and prescribe medical treatment, which can be harsh. When the desperate patient is unable to tolerate the treatment, they quit it like a bad habit—oftentimes without the support of the healthcare worker. The sudden cessation of treatment leads to new and worsening symptoms that the medical provider attributes to their unchallengeable diagnosis, when in reality the problems are treatment-induced. The patient spirals downward, while the doctor blames their demise on not following strict medical orders. If only people knew to exercise a great deal of wariness when dealing with healthcare "experts," they'd suffer a lot less!

Medical students are frankly told,

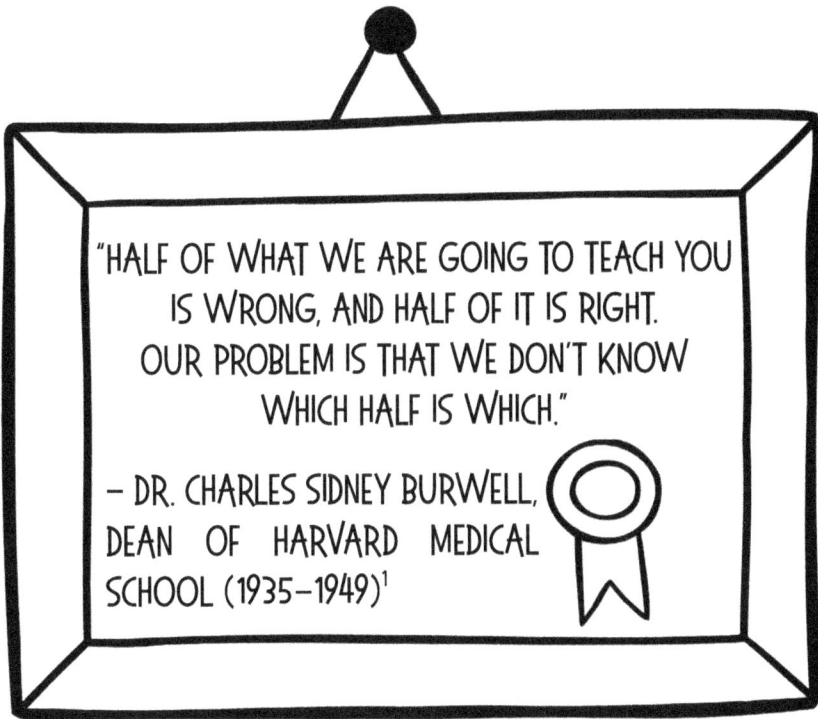

"HALF OF WHAT WE ARE GOING TO TEACH YOU IS WRONG, AND HALF OF IT IS RIGHT. OUR PROBLEM IS THAT WE DON'T KNOW WHICH HALF IS WHICH."

– DR. CHARLES SIDNEY BURWELL, DEAN OF HARVARD MEDICAL SCHOOL (1935–1949)[1]

How reassuring is this? If everything a doctor knows they learned in medical school, theoretically, that means half of everything they tell you about YOUR health is wrong! Add to that equation the element of human fallibility and a doctor likely knows a whole lot less than they claim to know. Taking continuing medical education (CME) is helpful to stay abreast of rapid advances in medicine; however, what Dr. Burwell said in his 1944 address to Harvard's Medical School students likely applies to CME too. This is why it's beneficial that patients cast their net wide rather than rely on a single healthcare resource for the right answers.

Society views doctors as walking medical encyclopedias, which is why every consumer-oriented health article starts or ends with, "Ask your doctor." If doctors have all the important answers, why are so many people sick and struggling? Even after 2,000 years of medicine, since the time of the ancient Greeks, the understanding of what ails and cures humans is still incomplete and evolving. The complexity of the human condition is too nuanced for professionals in lab coats and green scrubs to fully comprehend.

If patients didn't consider medical providers to be their sole saviors, they'd probably integrate the overabundance of accessible health resources into their daily lives to improve their overall well-being. Do you give your mechanic ultimate say over your car? Or are you careful how you accelerate, brake, and top up fluids in between service appointments? In the same way, patients have a degree of responsibility over the health of their body and mind.

Both sides would benefit in taking the unhealthy pressure off. The perception of the US healthcare industry demands a rehaul—or perhaps regular wellness checks.

2

Charting a New Healthcare Path

When you begin your healthcare journey, or if you're smack in the middle of it, a support crew helps you navigate around the rough patches, avoid falling into the terrifying abyss, and find health and safety.

Patients can round up a slew of health resources to form a tried-and-true support circle.

CONSUMER HEALTH WEBSITES

Credible health websites present current, balanced facts supported by scientific evidence and are written or reviewed by a licensed health professional.

They are consumer-oriented, meaning they do not require painful, time-consuming deciphering and do not convey important health information via medical gobbledygook (intelligible primarily by the healthcare professional species).

PATIENT SUPPORT GROUPS

Health woes shared are health woes halved.

Thus enters big-hearted patient support groups. Comprised of members waging war against a common health dilemma, patient support groups are sympathetic gatherings where health stories are swapped, coping tips are shared, and encouragement is freely given.

Patients join support groups to discuss chronic pain, heart disease, as well as Gaucher Disease, Sjogren's, and other conditions hard to roll off your tongue. Given there's a support group for Hidradenitis Suppurativa, patients can find a support group for almost any illness under the sun.

With the doors always open, in-person and online patient support groups dispel the isolation patients feel and forge a healing sense of community—without the deafening war cries.

ONLINE PATIENT FORUMS

Discussions of health experiences on online forums are potential goldmines for patients digging for affirmation of their experiences. Patients across continents gather in forums to share personal health stories, which often validate baffling symptoms.

Public forum answers to questions, like, "Is it diabetes or am I paranoid?" receive answers with a degree of accuracy on par with a doctor's.[1] However, physicians likely give the more complete answer.[1]

Doctors agree most information on discussion forums are "of reasonably good quality."[1] The small amount of low-quality information should be weeded out with the shrewdness of a gardener in claw gloves.[1]

The value of forums lies in a patient's lived experience versus a doctor's superficial textbook knowledge. A patient's intimate awareness of Auto-Brewery Syndrome symptoms that drag them through hell and back daily hold equivalent or superior value to a doctor's awareness of Auto-Brewery Syndrome symptoms learned about in a one-hour medical lecture from the comfort of an ergonomic chair.

As with all efforts to survive, exercising judicious caution while visiting online forums is a means of self-preservation.

PHARMACISTS

When a time-strapped physician doesn't tell you how you're expected to swallow that horse pill, a pharmacist comes to the rescue. The spectacled professional in white advises on the availability of chewable forms or whether it's safe for the monster drug to be crushed into applesauce or some other bland, mushy substance that makes you ask, "Why is this food?"[2]

Pharmacists serve as flavor specialists, too, capable of turning foul-tasting liquid prescriptions into palatable versions that don't do the wicked Samba Roll on your delicate tastebuds.

Offering advice on supplements to food and drug interactions, pharmacists are accessible resources to keep in your medicine cabinet. If they really don't want to be in there, just give them a call instead.

HEALTHCARE APPS

Modern technology is a boon for patients on the quest for health. Apps implore users to leverage their impressive monitoring capabilities and track fitness, weight, foods, as well as more detailed biomarkers of personal health, such as blood pressure and blood sugar.

Apps remind the forgetful to take medications on time and the obliviously parched to hydrate throughout the day. Log symptoms into symptom loggers to share with a medical provider.

While apps prove handy, overdependency can spur anxiety or guilt when patients miss a workout or are just a few pounds shy of their weight goals. Balanced use of apps, as with any health tools, creates more harmony and less agony.

Reducing agony—is there an app for that?

THIS JOURNAL

While intended to be helpful, this journal does not purport to have the answers in the vast field of ever-evolving medicine. Any answers are yours, scribbled in upon conscious self-assessment.

The journal asks some thought-provoking questions but not all thought-provoking questions. It provides some current medical facts but not all current medical facts. In short, it's among the countless incomprehensive resources that gloriously fail to provide thorough answers to all our burning questions, like, "What's that weird bump?" or "Why does that burn?" or "Should that be there?"

Patients can, however, consider its content and their own in consultation with a provider to arrive at the best healthcare decisions themselves—decisions that may be right today but not tomorrow, perhaps this hour but not the next. That's the lightning speed at which medicine advances. Thunderstruck?

YOUR TRUSTED RESOURCES

Today's patients aren't bound to one medical professional with limited availability and expertise. Rather, when they need healthcare most, a multitude of resources are at their fingertips to help them thrive.

Organize your most trusted personal healthcare resources.

Trusted Resource #1

_____

Trusted Resource #2

_____

Trusted Resource #3

_____

Trusted Resource #4

_____

Trusted Resource #5

_____

Trusted Resource #6

_____

Trusted Resource #7

_____

Trusted Resource #8

_____

Trusted Resource #9

_____

3

Patient (AKA Human) Liberties

Each person who receives medical care has a series of both human and patient rights. Among the many rights not to be trampled upon are the following five:

ALL PATIENTS HAVE THE RIGHT TO BE TREATED WITH DIGNITY BY MEDICAL PROFESSIONALS.[1]

This means being regarded as a capable individual, whether healthy as a horse or diagnosed with a socially stigmatized medical condition. No one chooses their illness. If we had dibs, we'd pick something nonfatal, causing minimal annoyance, and over in a split-second.

ALL PATIENTS HAVE THE RIGHT TO RECEIVE INFORMATION ABOUT PROPOSED TREATMENTS, THEIR BENEFITS, RISKS, AND COSTS, AS WELL AS INFORMATION ABOUT ANY RISKS OF DECLINING SUCH TREATMENTS.[1]

ALL PATIENTS HAVE THE RIGHT TO RECEIVE THE HEALTHCARE EXPERT'S GUIDANCE BASED ON "OBJECTIVE PROFESSIONAL JUDGMENT."[1]

Would you prefer a subjective "maybe-this'll-work" treatment or a clear course of action tested and proven to yield health benefits?

ALL PATIENTS HAVE THE RIGHT TO ASK THE PROVIDER QUESTIONS ABOUT THEIR CARE AND RECEIVE ANSWERS.[2]

This includes clarifying doubts until confident and not leaving the medical office (barricading if necessary) until questions are satisfactorily answered. Too many things can go wrong when pharmaceutical-happy physicians and scalpel-happy surgeons prescribe excessive or unnecessary care, which are often the culprit behind the onset of appalling new health concerns.

MEDICAL PROVIDERS MAY MAKE TREATMENT RECOMMENDATIONS— BUT PATIENTS OF SOUND MIND HAVE THE RIGHT TO MAKE THE FINAL DECISIONS REGARDING THEIR HEALTHCARE.[1]

This means they have the human and patient rights to accept care and refuse unwanted medical intervention and treatment.

Patients empower themselves by knowing and exercising their rights when grappling with the for-profit healthcare system that has a tendency to step on the toes of the unsuspecting. Avoid risking the torment of a stubbed toe—or worse!

EXERCISE YOUR RIGHTS.

TREADMILL NOT REQUIRED!

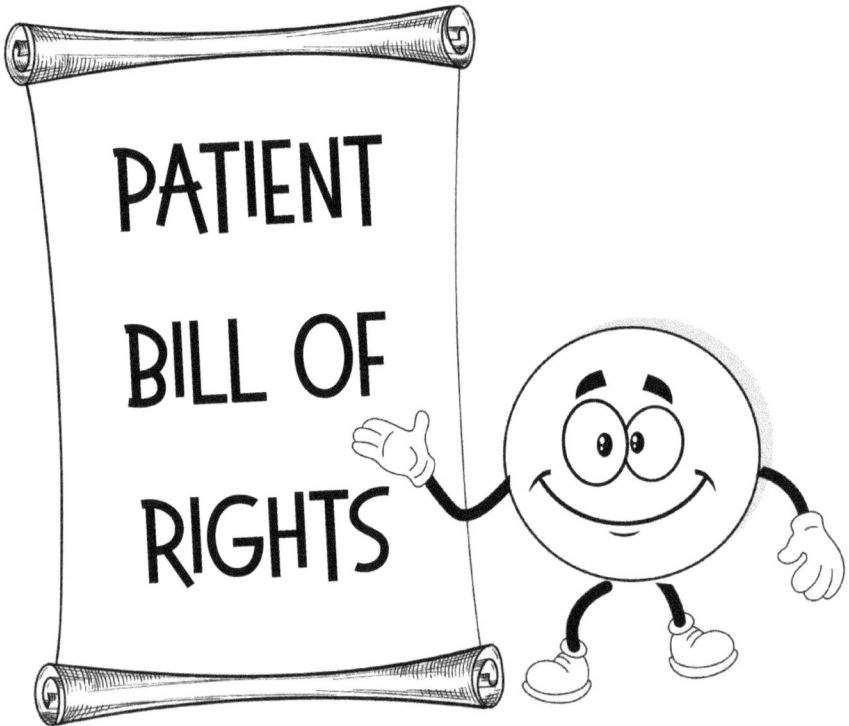

PATIENT BILL OF RIGHTS

4

Provider Examination

Not everyone goes into healthcare with the magnanimous intent to alleviate human pain and suffering. A few do enter the profession with noble intentions. But many choose the medical field for the wealth and status it brings. Doctors are still the highest-paid professionals in the nation, even taking the top rank over upstanding professional cuddlers and line standers.

Being a healthcare provider is like repairing vehicles. Except in the case of healthcare, the practitioner's job is to try to fix your body—unlike cars, there are no guarantees regarding the human machine. When a cure isn't available, at a minimum, the duties of a healthcare worker are to treat patients with active care, dignity, and compassion—which in themselves can be remarkably healing.

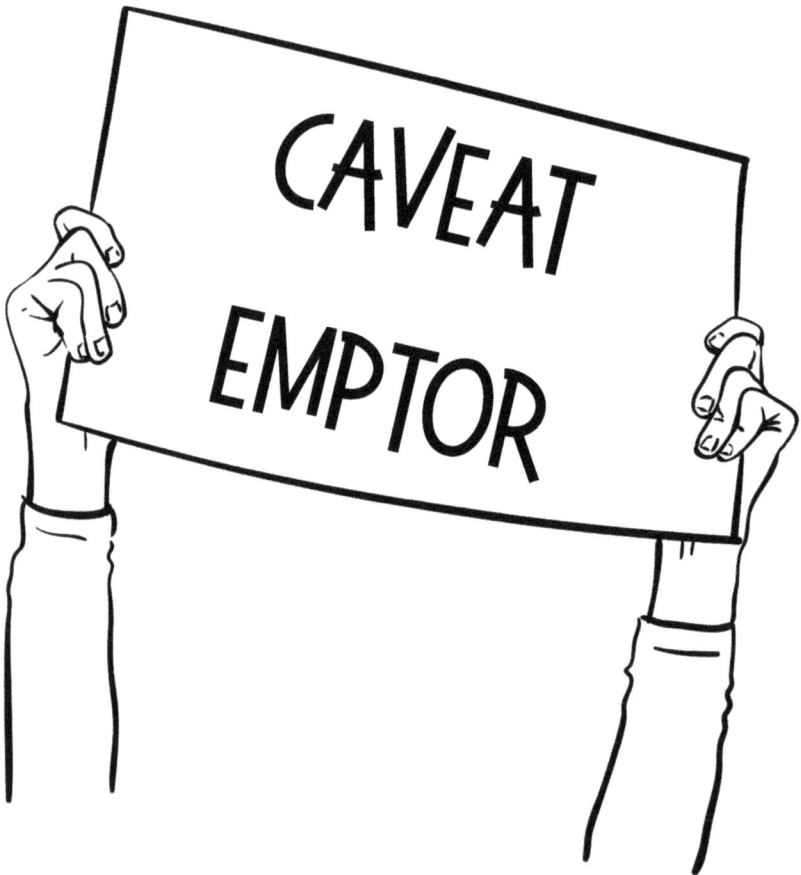

SURGEON FOR HIRE!

OPTOMETRIST FOR HIRE!

DOCTOR FOR HIRE!

DENTIST FOR HIRE!

NURSE FOR HIRE!

CAVEAT EMPTOR

COMPASSION

Many doctors are filled with years of accumulated medical textbook knowledge that compassion for the human condition is a sliver in their professional toolkit. Patients are sometimes treated like quick science experiments rather than vulnerable human beings with thoughts, feelings, and the capacity to suffer.

In defense of medical professionals, compassion burnout in the healthcare field is real. After all, who wants to listen to patients' complaints all day long, five days a week?

"Doc, my knee hurts."

"Doctor, the side effects are awful."

Or the complaint that bruises their ego: "Doctor, I think you've given me the wrong diagnosis."

How dare a sick, little patient challenge a powerful doctor who's gone through several rigorous years of medical school, enjoys the support of his esteemed colleagues, and hangs a framed diploma on his wall?

Patients have the right to question a diagnosis when doubts arise. The patient's lived experience—feeling, managing, and coping with their symptoms every day—surpasses any medical handbook and affirms the patient's authority over their well-being. The doctor merely has superficial textbook or observational knowledge. The depth of difference is profound.

Every patient should be awarded a diploma, with distinction, that rivals a doctor's medical diploma.

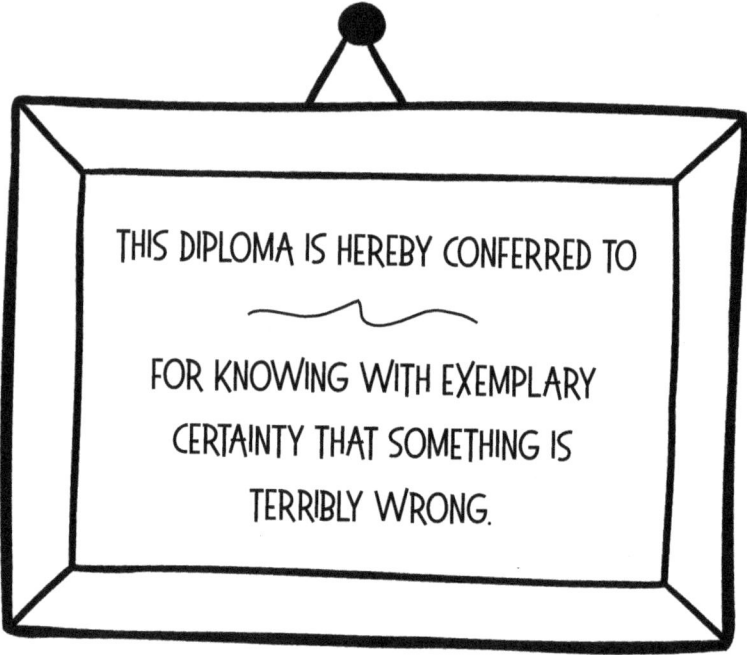

THIS DIPLOMA IS HEREBY CONFERRED TO

FOR KNOWING WITH EXEMPLARY CERTAINTY THAT SOMETHING IS TERRIBLY WRONG.

versus

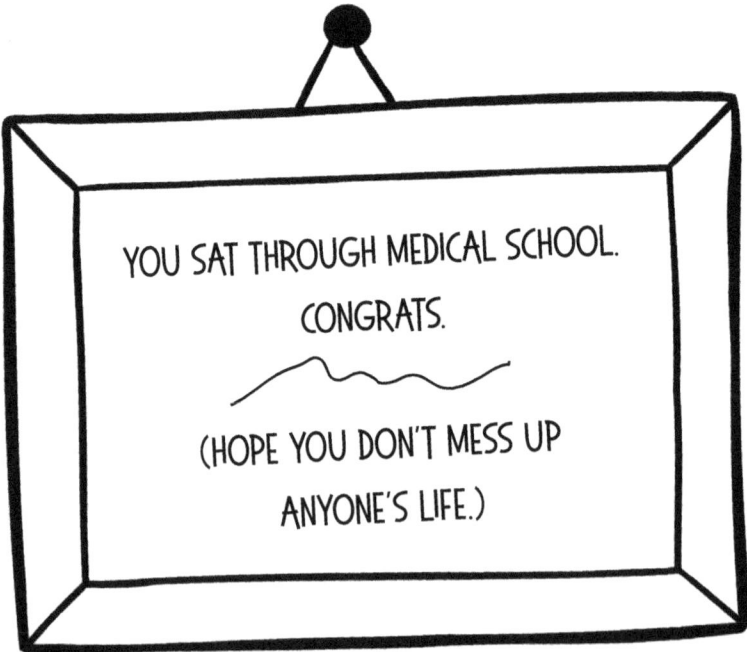

YOU SAT THROUGH MEDICAL SCHOOL. CONGRATS.

(HOPE YOU DON'T MESS UP ANYONE'S LIFE.)

But just as real are patients who find doctors conscientious enough to know how to avert professional burnout while still delivering consistent, quality care. Fortunate is the patient whose doctor balances medical skill with compassion.

QUALITY OF VISIT

Doctors endure four grueling years of medical school plus three or more years in residency under an insufferable chief resident and perhaps a few additional years in a fellowship program only to spend fifteen minutes with the patient and charge $300 on top of it. Despite the dedicated training to learn to help patients, medical providers are in and out of the exam room in a jiffy, some even adding a dose of insulting arrogance to their highly sought-after yet at times substandard services.

Every patient is the Chief Executive Officer (CEO) of their health enterprise (consisting of body, mind, and spirit). It's vital they hire a team to ensure this enterprise prospers. A patient's only opportunity to interview a new healthcare provider is during the first appointment.

List your top three current health goals.

1. _____

2. _____

3. _____

Describe four qualities you seek in a healthcare practitioner.

1. _____

2. _____

3. _____

4. _____

Does your provider actively listen to your health concerns?

_____

_____

_____

Do you feel you can communicate honestly?

_____

_____

_____

Describe the provider's demeanor. Reasonable, unchallengeable, something else? How do you foresee this affecting your care?

_____

_____

_____

_____

_____

Do you believe this professional will help you achieve your health objectives? Why or why not?

_____

_____

_____

_____

_____

"DOC, I'M HERE FOR A REFILL."

"TO GET A REFILL, YOU MUST SEE ME THIRTEEN TIMES A YEAR AND TAKE THIS PRICEY EXERCISE STRESS TEST."

"BUT THIRTEEN? WHY?"

"OTHERWISE MY PATIENTS WOULDN'T SEE ME. HOW DO YOU EXPECT ME TO PAY MY BILLS?"

$700 WORTH OF OUT-OF-POCKET PATIENT TEST EXPENSES LATER...

"UM, DOC, YOU COULD'VE JUST TOLD ME TO LOSE A FEW POUNDS."

"SHUSH! I AM YOUR MASTER. YOU DO WHAT I SAY!"

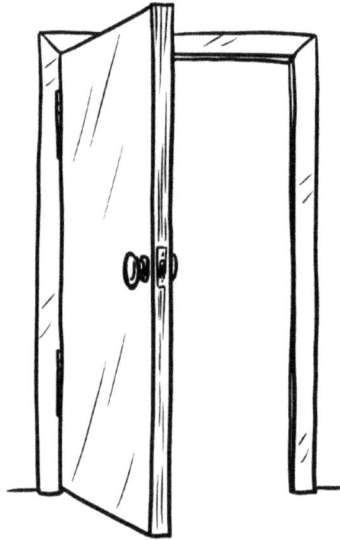

DR. MACHIAVELLIANA

Does your provider use manipulation tactics?

_____

_____

_____

Some providers are quick to prescribe harsh, expensive treatments required to jump over multiple insurance hurdles—when equally effective, less costly, and accessible over-the-counter remedies without disastrous side effects are available immediately.

What drives their reckless ambition to overprescribe? It's an unerring case of whydunit. Whoever solves it deserves to be inducted into the Patient Advocate Hall of Fame for giving the greatest health benefits to humankind, advancing wellness despite the health industry's injurious effects, and be given recognition for a transformative discovery that saves patients from a wretched quality of life.

Perhaps health workers should follow this
rudimentary formula:

FEAR OF UNDERPRESCRIBING X FEAR OF OVERPRESCRIBING = CONFIDENCE IN CORRECTLY PRESCRIBING

Both negative fears cancel each other out, resulting in positive
patient outcomes.

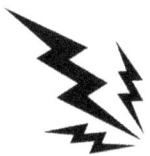

I WIELD THE REMARKABLE SUPERPOWER TO PRESCRIBE. IT DOMINATES OVER ALL GOOD SENSE!

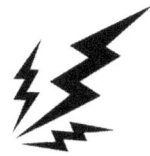

If the health worker prescribes treatment, do you believe it is excessive, just right, or not enough?

_____

_____

_____

_____

_____

Does your doctor pile upon remedies without addressing the root cause of the issue, such as treatment side effects, stress, or lifestyle factors?

_____

_____

_____

_____

_____

Do you leave the visit with an actionable care plan or a resolution of your health concerns?

_____

_____

_____

_____

_____

_____

_____

_____

_____

As in any successful enterprise, conducting periodic reevaluations of a health expert ensures they continue to fulfill care objectives. Working with a compatible provider improves the course of a patient's healthcare journey—like cheese enhances crackers, except when the cheese is rancid.

List three pros and cons of staying with your current health provider.

Pros (established trust, familiarity with health?):

1. _____

2. _____

3. _____

Cons (possibility of continuing a misdiagnosis, older treatment options?):

1. _____

2. _____

3. _____

List three pros and cons of switching to a new provider.

Pros (possibility of a new diagnosis, more advanced or gentler treatments?):

1. _____

2. _____

3. _____

Cons (a need to rebuild trust and health history?):

1. _____

2. _____

3. _____

A patient-doctor relationship is built on mutual respect and cooperation. It's a partnership in working toward the same goals: optimal patient health and satisfaction.

PATIENTS OFTEN STAY WITH THE SAME PROVIDER FOR CONTINUITY OF CARE. BUT FOR UNINFORMED PATIENTS, IT CREATES A RISK FOR CONTINUITY OF CARELESSNESS.

5

Symptom ID

You've got to *help* your provider help you.

Uttering, "Doc, my arm hurts," might be met with a dumbfounded stare.

Instead saying, "Doctor, I feel pain in my inner elbow when I golf for an hour every day," is far more precise and likely to achieve desirable results. But to get to a point of exactness, the patient must do their part. This is where patient resources, like this journal, come in handy.

It's important to distinguish between an inherent medical condition and temporary poor health caused by modifiable factors, such as environment, medications, and stress, among others. Patients can be in good health one week, but a series of off days or stressful event takes a toll on their well-being the next.

Do you enjoy a clean bill of health?

_____

_____

_____

_____

_____

Or does your body signal that something is wrong?

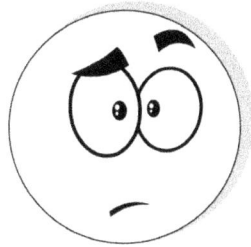

_____

_____

____ _____

_____

_____

_____

If so, what bothersome symptoms do you experience?

_____

_____

_____

_____

_____

How often do you experience these symptoms?

_____

_____

_____

_____

_____

Are these symptoms new or ongoing? If new, when did they start?

_____

_____

_____

_____

If ongoing, how many days, weeks, months, or years have you been experiencing them?

_____

_____

_____

_____

_____

What, if anything, relieves these symptoms?

_____

_____

_____

_____

What do you attribute these symptoms to? An injury, illness, food, medication, activity, stress, something else?

_____

_____

_____

_____

_____

What do you notice triggers your symptoms?

_____

_____

_____

_____

_____

Based on what triggers your symptoms, do you believe your condition can be alleviated with lifestyle modifications, such as stress management, nutrition, or exercise?

_____

_____

_____

_____

_____

Or do you think you'd benefit from medical treatment, like physical therapy, medication, or surgery?

_____

_____

_____

_____

_____

Are you willing to discuss these possibilities with your healthcare provider?

_____

_____

_____

_____

_____

6

Sizing Up a Diagnosis

A medical diagnosis is life-changing—that's why it should be dead-on. The thorny part is that not all ailments are diagnosed based on objective test results. Some diagnoses stem from a doctor's subjective interpretation—which can introduce human inaccuracies. Chronic fatigue, mental health conditions, and autism, for example, are tricky to nail down.[1, 2] Correctly diagnosing complex illnesses like these and others can be a slow-as-molasses process, taking months or sometimes years.[3] But it brings sweet relief when a diagnosis is finally spot-on.

Understanding symptoms and communicating them to a healthcare professional can lead to a right diagnosis and hopefully sooner. A proper diagnosis is critical, as it guides the course of treatment. If a provider says that the diagnosis doesn't matter only the symptoms, it's a red flag. No patient wants to be put on the wrong drug or endure long-term, unnecessary, and potentially harmful treatments causing debilitating side effects—for a condition they don't have. Conversely, an accurate diagnosis puts patients on the path to improved well-being and helps them make the right healthcare calls.

What diagnosis were you given?

_____

_____

_____

What tests did the healthcare worker perform to arrive at this diagnosis? Physical exam, bloodwork, neurological test, biopsy, something else?

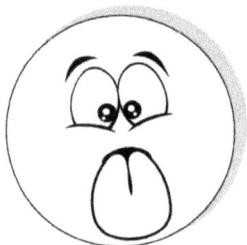

_____

_____

_____

_____

Did the provider take a medical history (to determine allergies, lifestyle, past illnesses) and a family history (to look for genetic patterns and conditions)?

_____

_____

_____

_____

_____

Do you have a family history of this condition?

_____

_____

_____

_____

_____

Did you speak with other patients or visit forums geared toward those with the same condition? If so, what similarities or dissimilarities did you uncover?

SIMILARITIES

_____

_____

_____

_____

DISSIMILARITIES

_____

_____

_____

_____

If you performed research about this condition, list your top three authoritative resources. What did you learn?

1. _____

2. _____

3. _____

Helpful Information Learned:

_____

_____

_____

_____

_____

_____

_____

Based on the symptoms you experience, speaking with other patients, and/or performing research, do you feel this diagnosis is accurate? Why or why not?

_____

_____

_____

_____

_____

Did you or will you seek a second opinion if you have doubts or disagree?

_____

_____

_____

_____

If you sought a second opinion, list the diagnosis.

_____

_____

_____

Do you agree with the second-opinion diagnosis? Why or why not?

_____

_____

_____

_____

_____

_____

A diagnosis isn't always carved in stone. When the unforeseeable occurs, it can change. An illness resolves out of the blue. New technologies, like DNA scanning, give health experts mind-blowing insights.[4] Pioneering treatments drop. Or perplexing symptoms become clear as day as medicine evolves, leading to a different diagnosis altogether.

A second opinion from another medical expert offers a new perspective, like a refreshing hike across a moon-like landscape produces clarity and peace of mind—and a bit of the surreal.

MISDIAGNOSES

Mosquitoes and misdiagnoses are deadly yet terribly common—bringing discomfort and disruption to the lives of millions of Americans each year. The sum of annual known medical misdiagnoses over a mere 28.5 years equals the current population of the entire country.

And like mosquitoes, misdiagnoses cause unnecessary suffering, a miserable quality of life, and sometimes suck the life right out of the patient.

Whether a doctor fails to thoroughly examine symptoms—and all possible causes—before giving a potentially life-shattering diagnosis because...

they don't have the time ("Your fifteen minutes are up.")

or...

they don't want to ("Who's the doctor here?")

or...

they don't feel the need to ("100% of what they teach us in medical school is correct.")

...it's critical that patients incorporate the abundance of verifiable health resources into their care and be an active participant in their well-being.

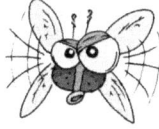

"DOCTOR, I THINK I HAVE SPOTS."

"I SEE STRIPES."

"UM..."

"WHAT DID YOUR PREVIOUS DOCTOR SAY?"

"UH, SHE SAID STRIPES."

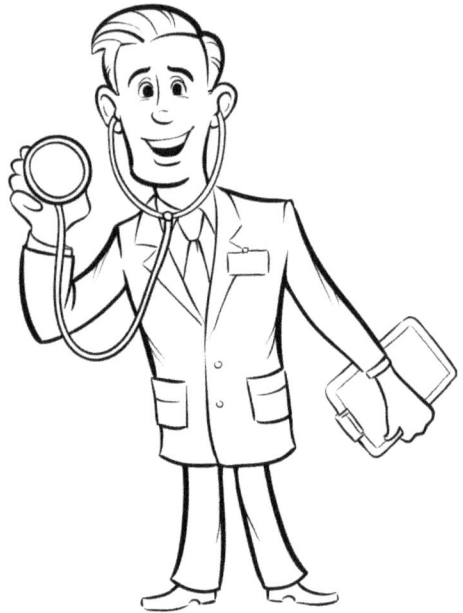

"IF MY ESTEEMED COLLEAGUE SAID STRIPES, IT'S STRIPES! WE GRADUATED MEDICAL SCHOOL, THE PINNACLE OF ACHIEVEMENT. WE KNOW SPOTS FROM STRIPES! I'M WRITING YOU A SCRIPT FOR STRIPES."

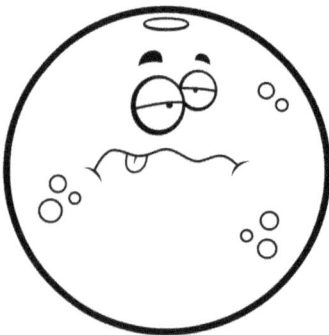

"BUT......SPOTS."

"STRIPES!"

7

Kicking Off a Medication Regimen

Every patient who receives medical treatment has the right to be informed of its risks, benefits, and potential side effects.[1] Monitoring for side effects is a critical part of a health provider's responsibility, and failure to do so can lead to devastating patient outcomes. At the same time, clinicians cannot adjust medications or dosages unless they are aware of the side effects the patient experiences.

Sometimes medication side effects are subtle or develop so gradually that the patient is unaware that the drug is responsible. Rather, it's not uncommon for patients to attribute intolerable side effects to symptoms of their health condition. This is why medication monitoring by a healthcare provider is crucial to preventing harmful effects in patients.

Before taking a medication, it's highly beneficial to gain a clear understanding of its purpose, how it improves symptoms, and learn what it should do for you. Certain medicines are dicey for particular demographics, like the elderly who might resort to the American Geriatric Society Beers Criteria to search for drugs risky for their age group.

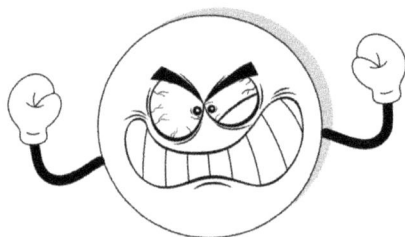

Various medicines are bullies. They literally beat you up—leaving you disoriented, nauseous, and in worse condition than before starting them. Other medications help you feel better, like a steady friend when you need her most. Listening to how the body reacts helps differentiate foe from friend.

A tiny, harmless-looking pill has the immense power to alter body chemistry, arguably similar to changing an innocent bat into

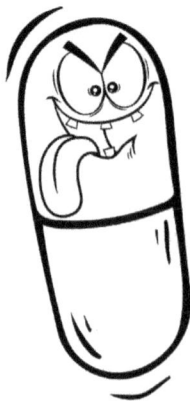

a blood-thirsty vampire on a ravenous midnight prowl or a best bud into a night-stalking werewolf howling at the full moon in a fit of insanity. Patients who tread carefully when dealing with medications avoid petrifying transformations.

What medication are you being prescribed?

_____

_____

_____

What is the dose?

_____

_____

_____

List the date you started this drug.

_____

_____

_____

What is the purpose of taking this medication?

_____

_____

_____

_____

How will this medicine help your symptoms?

_____

_____

_____

_____

_____

Do you notice any benefits upon starting this drug?

_____

_____

_____

_____

Per the prescriber, how many days, weeks, or months before you can expect to feel better?

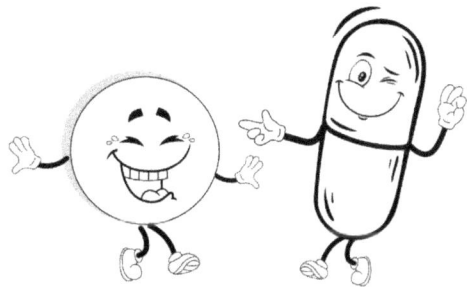

_____

_____

_____

_____

_____

What are the prescriber's instructions on how to take this medication (eg, with or without food), its duration (eg, days, weeks, months), and frequency (eg, number of times per day)?

_____

_____

_____

_____

If the physician did not give clear instructions, did you consult a pharmacist or nurse? What are their instructions?

_____

_____

_____

_____

_____

MEDICATION SIDE EFFECTS

Did the prescriber inform you of possible medication side effects?
If so, list them.

_____

_____

_____

_____

Does your provider actively monitor for side effects (eg, symptom
reviews, physical exams, blood tests)?

_____

_____

_____

_____

Do you notice any new side effects upon starting the drug? If so, describe what you experience.

_____

_____

Side Effects Day 1: _____

Side Effects Day 2: _____

Side Effects Day 3: _____

Side Effects Day 4: _____

Side Effects Day 5: _____

Side Effect Day 6: _____

Side Effects Day 7: _____

How long have you been experiencing these side effects?

_____

_____

_____

Are these side effects gradually diminishing as your body adjusts to the medicine?

_____

_____

_____

If the side effects are bothersome, when will you discuss them with the prescriber?

_____

_____

MEDICATION INTERACTIONS

Are you taking other prescription medicines, supplements, vitamins, or herbal medicines? If so, list them and their doses.

Prescription Medicines and Doses:

_____

_____

Supplements and Doses:

_____

_____

Vitamins and Doses:

_____

_____

Herbal Medicines and Doses:

_____

_____

Some medications (even over-the-counter drugs you thought were as nice as your neighbors) don't play well with others.

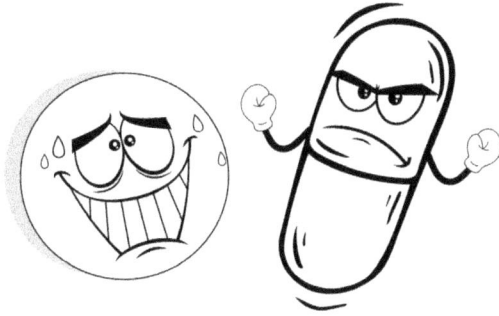

Note any possible medication interactions you discussed with the healthcare provider.

_____

_____

_____

_____

_____

_____

_____

MEDICATION REVIEWS

Periodic medication reviews allow prescribers to assess whether a medication should be continued, stopped, or adjusted. A patient's condition may change over time, making reviews highly beneficial.

Questions to ask before starting a drug regimen include...

1. What are the long-term effects of this medicine?

2. Does the medication cause dependency?

3. Will I develop a tolerance to this drug (requiring higher doses to stay effective)?

4. Is routine therapeutic drug monitoring (such as labs) necessary?

And during a medication review...

1. Do I still need to take this medicine?

When is your next medication review?

_____

What questions do you have for your prescriber?

Question 1: _____

_____

Question 2: _____

_____

Question 3: _____

_____

Question 4: _____

_____

8

Calling a Medication Quits

It's generally advised to never abruptly stop a medication without consulting a healthcare provider. Suddenly stopping a prescription drug can cause severe withdrawal symptoms and, depending on the medication, more serious health problems than before starting it.[1]

This warning applies to not only medications in pill form but also prescription creams, like topical steroids, patches, and liquid solutions.

"WHAT? YOU'RE BREAKING UP WITH ME AFTER ALL THIS TIME? THIS CALLS FOR REVENGE!"

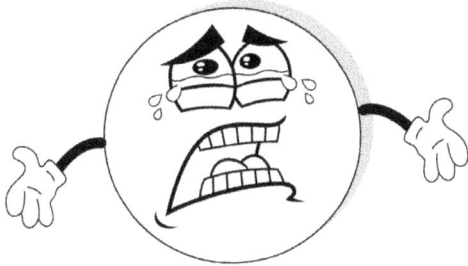

Tapering is a process of gradually reducing a medication dose to give the body time to adjust and lessen withdrawal symptoms.

Are you considering stopping a medication?

_____

_____

What is the medication and the dose?

_____

_____

List the primary reason you wish to stop this drug.

_____

_____

_____

Have you discussed tapering with the prescriber? If so, what are their tapering instructions?

_____

_____

_____

If you have questions about the tapering plan, what does the doctor, nurse, or pharmacist recommended?

_____

_____

_____

COMPOUND PHARMACIES

Accredited pharmacies can compound medications, which means creating smaller, custom doses to help patients safely taper off a medicine. Patients usually need to provide the compound pharmacy with a prescription from their healthcare provider for the smaller dose to start the process. Compounded drugs, however, are not approved by the Food and Drug Administration (FDA).[2]

9

Going Under the Knife

In the Golden Age of American Capitalism, Dr. Paul Hawley, Director of American College of Surgeons, revealed, "The public would be shocked if it knew the amount of unnecessary surgery performed..."[1]

Today's surgeons performing needless surgeries still show no signs of pulling in the horns in the Wild West of the operating room.

"YEEHAW!"

"I DON'T HAVE ANY FINANCIAL INCENTIVES."

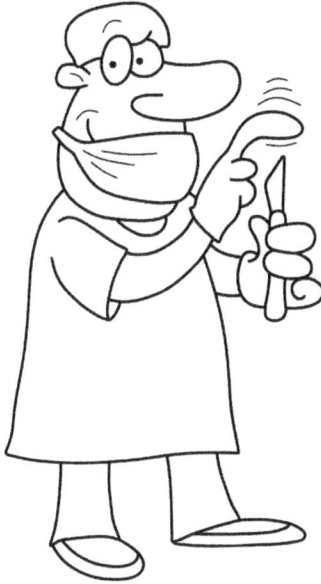

The decision to undergo elective surgery is made upon careful deliberation of whether it's necessary and if the benefits outweigh the risks. It's not uncommon for the thousands of unnecessary surgeries performed each year to offer little if any benefit while carrying high risk of complications.[1]

For instance, slightly more than half of total knee replacement patients feel some level of regret, whether due to higher pain or decreased mobility, in the aftermath of the procedure.[2]

49% feel no regret[2]

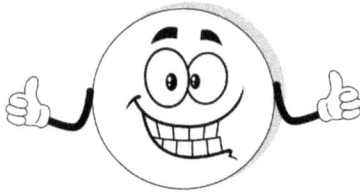

25% feel a little regret[2]

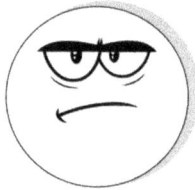

26% feel a whole lot of regret[2]

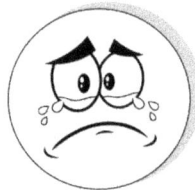

Yet surgery can prevent complications.

"WELL, THIS BROKEN BONE WON'T FIX ITSELF."

"WHY DOES THAT LARGE MOLE KEEP CHANGING SHAPE?"

Are you considering surgery?

_____

_____

What are the proposed benefits of the surgical procedure?

_____

_____

_____

_____

What are the risks associated with the operation?

_____

_____

_____

_____

Do the benefits outweigh the risks?

_____

_____

_____

_____

_____

_____

Will you require additional surgeries in the future?

_____

_____

_____

_____

What can you expect during the surgical recovery phase?

_____

_____

_____

_____

_____

How do you define surgical "success"? Long-term pain relief, improved motion, something else?

_____

_____

_____

_____

_____

What have you learned about the regret and success rates of other surgical patients?

REGRET RATE: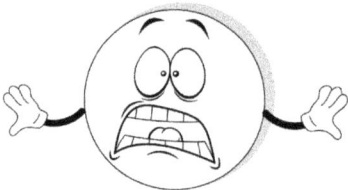

_____

_____

_____

_____

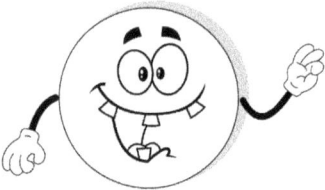 SUCCESS RATE:

_____

_____

_____

_____

How do you expect the surgery to impact you long-term (one, two, or five years)?

_____

_____

_____

_____

_____

_____

_____

_____

_____

_____

10

Less-Squeamish (Non-Surgical) Options

In lieu of costly, high-risk elective surgeries without a 100% guarantee of lifelong relief from pain, patients might explore less expensive, non-invasive treatment options.

Medical experts sometimes recommend a combination of non-surgical interventions to deliver better results.[1]

Physical Therapy[1]
MOVE THOSE MUSCLES!

Regenerative Medicine[1]
IN STEM CELL THERAPY YOUR OWN CELLS DO THE HEALING

Transcutaneous Electrical Nerve Stimulation[1]
ZAP CHRONIC PAIN WITH ELECTRICAL CURRENTS

Bracing[1]
NOTHING FEELS MORE RIGHT THAN PROPER ALIGNMENT

Injection Therapy[1]
HOPE YOU'RE NOT SCARED OF NEEDLES!

Hydrotherapy[1]
WHO DOESN'T LOVE SPLASHING IN WATER?

Creams and Patches[1]
A LITTLE PATCH COULDN'T HURT

Massage Therapy[1]
A RELAXING MASSAGE, ANYONE?

Anti-inflammatory Diet[1]
FRUITS AND VEGGIES EVERY DAY HELP KEEP SURGERY AWAY!

Are you exploring non-surgical approaches to healing?

_____

_____

If so, what surgical alternatives seem promising based on your symptoms, health goals, and discussions with your medical provider?

_____

_____

_____

_____

_____

_____

_____

11

Alt (Alternative) Medicine

Contemporary health treatments are driven by advances in medicine. But for thousands of years, alternative medicine has healed countless people or at least helped them manage their conditions. From ancient Chinese herbal medicines to 5,000-year-old Indian meditation practices, alternative treatments improve body, mind, and soul. Alternative medicine is gentler than conventional medicine without the damaging side effects, making it a desirable complement to traditional healthcare.[1]

Alternative medicine is an expansive field but includes these low-cost, accessible, and rather delightful forms of healing. In fact, many partake in their joyous aspects whether they are managing an illness or not!

ACUPUNCTURE

This Traditional Chinese Medicine is not for the squeamish around needles or those with certain health issues. But for the adventurous, inserting hair-thin needles into any of the body's 2,000 pressure points stimulates the nervous system and releases waves of feel-good chemicals.[2] It brings relief for arthritis, migraines, and anxiety, among other conditions.[2]

If you are considering acupuncture, have you discussed with your doctor whether it's safe for you?

_____

_____

_____

_____

Has your healthcare provider, friends, or family referred you to a licensed acupuncturist?

_____

MEDITATION

Kicking back and focusing thoughts are no sweat—with a little practice. Meditation doesn't require pricey gym memberships or embarrassing workout clothes and can be practiced despite the weather, even when it's raining frogs. Yet it helps control anxiety, reduce stress, improve sleep, and decrease high blood pressure.[3] Getting in the meditative zone also has the potential to lessen chronic pain.[3]

How would it feel to sit for 5 to 10 minutes a day, eyes closed, clearing the mind, and indulging in a state of relaxation and calm?

_____

_____

Can you gradually increase to 60 minutes of daily meditation for deeper health benefits?

_____

What is your least distracting place to meditate? In a quiet nook at home, next to a serene river, on a balcony to catch the sunrise?

_____

AROMATHERAPY

Scents take us back—or forward toward well-being. Aromatherapy harnesses the feel-good power of essential oils, obtained from herbs. Inhaling these oils rouses the olfactory system and puts patients on cloud nine with feelings, like calm or comfort.[4]

Aromatherapy is thought to help improve insomnia (cinnamon essential oil), pain (lavender essential oil), nausea (peppermint essential oil), and anxiety (chamomile essential oil), among other conditions.[4]

Are you allergic to essential oils? The sensitive may want to dodge certain essential oils, like cinnamon bark, tea tree, and clove, which tend to be triggering.[5]

_____

Are you choosing pure essential oils?

_____

Tips include

A LABEL CONTAINING THE LATIN PLANT NAME
BOTTLED IN DARK-COLORED GLASS
INDICATING 100% ESSENTIAL OIL (RATHER THAN SYNTHETIC
FRAGRANCE OIL)[6]

FOREST BATHING

Taking a dip in the forest stimulates all five senses, sending richly oxygenated air into the schnoz.[7] Forest bathing—spending a few hours in the midst of trees—is good for humans, reducing stress, depression, and blood pressure and improving sleep, among a winsome host of other sweet pickings.[7]

Forests live on one-third of the planet, giving the lucky few access. If you are among the other two-thirds, what would it feel like to stroll through a local park instead for a health boost?[7]

_____

_____

_____

_____

Are you willing to find a few hours regularly, like during day trips, to immerse yourself in nature and reap the full benefits? If not, even fifteen minutes counts.[7]

_____

SUNSHINE THERAPY

Sunlight—in sensible amounts—helps alleviate low back pain, depression, and other awful conditions.[8] Known as heliotherapy, sunshine therapy enhances the immune system, regulates sleep, and synthesizes vitamin D.[8]

Describe three activities you can do to increase your exposure to a healthy amount of direct sunlight.

OUTDOOR PILATES
BIRDWATCHING BY THE WINDOW
OPENING THE CURTAINS

1. _____

_____

2. _____

_____

3. _____

_____

Too much sun exposure is harmful. List 3 to 5 ways to protect yourself from the sun.

APPLY SUNSCREEN
SPORT SUNGLASSES AND A WIDE-BRIMMED HAT
LIMIT TIME IN THE SUN TO 10 TO 30 MINUTES PER DAY

1. _____

_____

2. _____

_____

3. _____

_____

4. _____

_____

5. _____

_____

12

Lifestyle Upgrades

The nuts and bolts of wellness rely upon common sense: eat right, exercise, and avoid unhealthy habits, like smoking, drinking excessively, and trekking inside active volcanos.

Although we know lifestyle, diet, and exercise are foundations of good health, sometimes these factors play little role in longevity or overall well-being. George Burns, the legendary American actor, lived to be one hundred while smoking cigars (but never inhaling), drinking martinis and scotch, and eating fried foods.[1] Yet it's equally surprising when an adult who plays weekly tennis and conscientiously eats a heart-healthy diet collapses with a heart attack at a ripe young age.

The human body is a conundrum.

The late George Burns is the exception. More often than not, however, a sedentary lifestyle, smoking, and gorging on a daily diet of ultra-processed foods puts folks on a collision course with disease.

When illness strikes, patients turn to health practitioners—the gatekeepers to vital medical treatments.

But not all are obligated to pass through these gates heavily guarded by doctors' orders, insurance companies, and prescriptive authority. Instead, many people bypass them altogether by helping prevent illness with lifestyle upgrades.

By making lifestyle enhancements, the chances of health roll in their favor.

EATING RIGHT AND HYDRATING

Fruits, vegetables, whole grains, legumes, and lean proteins are packed with the vitamins and minerals bodies need to function optimally, boost the immune system, and strengthen muscles and bones.

Do you limit your daily intake of sugars, unhealthy fats, and salt?

_____

_____

_____

List your favorite healthy foods.

_____

_____

_____

_____

_____

Do you feed your body these regularly? If not, describe how you can incorporate them into meals.

_____

_____

_____

_____

_____

Up to sixty percent of the adult human body is water.[2] Humans are like walking fish. It's essential to stay hydrated so the body performs. Symptoms of dehydration, like dry skin, fatigue, and dizziness, can mimic certain health conditions.[3] At the moment of thirst, the body is starting to dehydrate.

List three ways you can hydrate throughout the day.

FLAVOR A PITCHER OF WATER WITH LEMON
EAT WATER-RICH FOODS
SET HYDRATION REMINDERS ON A PHONE

1. _____

_____

2. _____

_____

3. _____

_____

EXERCISING REGULARLY

Walking, bicycling, swimming, as well as playing with the grandkids and dancing like no one's watching, are valid, if not euphoric, forms of physical activity.

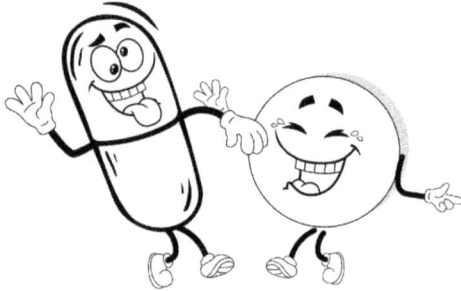

Conversely, those with the prestigious but slightly deadly title of desk jockey increase their chances of a reduced lifespan due to heart disease, cancer, and diabetes.[4] Sitting all day without periods of physical activity is remarkably dire for health.

If most days consist of parking yourself in one spot, list 3 to 4 ways you can break it up at regular intervals, like every hour.

1. _____

2. _____

3. _____

4. _____

Adults are generally recommended to exercise at least 150 minutes per week (eg, 30 minutes a day, 5 days a week).[5]

The more you exercise, the greater the health benefits.

EXORCISE DISEASE WITH EXERCISE!

How often do you exercise?

_____

_____

What physical activities do you enjoy?

_____

_____

_____

_____

_____

How do you feel after a bout of physical activity?

☐ STRONG
☐ HEALTHY
☐ VIBRANT

Something else?

_____

Does this motivate you to continue exercising?

_____

_____

_____

_____

_____

_____

GETTING QUALITY SLEEP

Sleep is an opportunity for the tired body to regenerate. It's also one of the few blissful hours when dreamers are chased by monstrous beetles, fly through the exosphere, or free fall through cumulus clouds. Who wouldn't awaken refreshed?

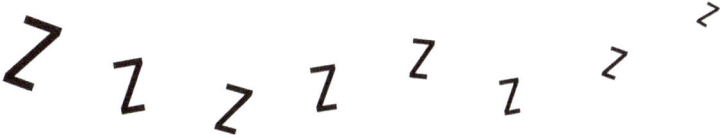

Z Z Z Z Z Z Z Z

At least seven hours of quality sleep are generally recommended for adults.

How many hours do you sleep each night?

_____

Do you sleep uninterrupted throughout the night? Or do you awaken periodically?

_____

_____

_____

_____

If you have trouble falling or staying asleep, what do you believe interferes with your sleep?

_____

_____

_____

List 3 to 4 adjustments you can make to promote better sleep quality.

GO TO BED AT THE SAME TIME EACH NIGHT
EXERCISE MORE
RESOLVE STRESS

1. _____

2. _____

3. _____

4. _____

MANAGING STRESS

Stress is a beast—and feeling it regularly feeds the growth of numerous problems, from cardiovascular disease to mental health issues and chronic fatigue.

Stress relievers include these four:

JOURNAL TO RELEASE PENT-UP EMOTIONS
CONFIDE IN A FRIEND
PRACTICE DEEP BREATHING
TAKE A STROLL TO CLEAR YOUR MIND AND GAIN
NEW PERSPECTIVE

List three ways you can minimize your stress levels starting today.

1. _____

_____

2. _____

_____

3. _____

_____

STAYING SOCIALLY ACTIVE

Loneliness not only feels like being caught in the suffocating grips of despair but is unfavorable to health. The chronically lonely increase their risks for early death, depression, and heart disease among other dreadful outcomes.[6]

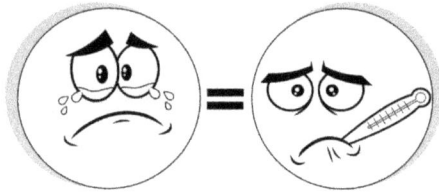

If you enjoy the company of others, do you maintain an active social life?

_____

_____

_____

_____

_____

If not, list three activities you can start tomorrow to feel more connected with others.

VOLUNTEER FOR A MEANINGFUL CAUSE
SPEND TIME WITH A PET
JOIN A GARDENING CLUB, BOOK CLUB, SQUIRREL CLUB...

1. _____

_____

2. _____

_____

3. _____

_____

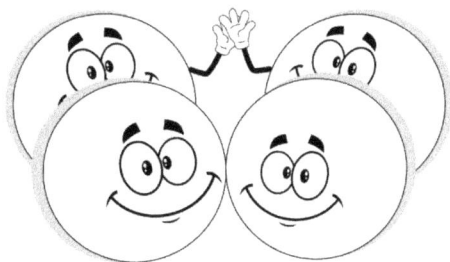

PURSUING HOBBIES

Whether you are passionate about duck herding, extreme ironing, or soap carving, hobbies improve life satisfaction. Participating in hobbies increases happiness, decreases stress, and fosters social connections.[7] Nothing builds friendships like extreme ironers ascending Scottish hills, paddling canoes, and meandering into caves—with a full-size ironing board in tow—and ironing. The awe doubles when the hobbyists show off a perfectly pressed shirt.

A LITTLE HAPPINESS A DAY KEEPS THE DOCTOR AWAY![8]

List the hobbies that renew your zest for life.

_____

_____

_____

_____

_____

_____

Do you actively participate in them? Why or why not?

_____

_____

_____

_____

If not, describe how you can adapt hobbies you once enjoyed so you pick them up again.

_____

_____

_____

_____

_____

13

The Boring-But-Necessary Medical Records Review

Subjective diagnoses should be noted as such in a patient's medical record since they are based on a doctor's interpretation rather than clear and accurate clinical data from test results. Human interpretation is often flawed. When a doctor or other healthcare practitioner provides a diagnosis that is based on subjective interpretation, it follows the patient to subsequent doctors, many of whom are reluctant to disagree with their medical colleagues—even if the diagnosis seems incorrect.

This herd mentality among medical workers comes at the patient's expense. Patients who lack knowledge may hesitatingly accept the wrong diagnosis or fear to speak up due to the intimidating authority of health professionals. The mistaken diagnosis perpetuates, and the patient ends up with unnecessary treatment that is oftentimes more harmful than helpful. Their symptoms do not improve, or the treatment causes more health problems that they attribute to this erroneous medical condition they are convinced to believe they have.

Patients are encouraged to review their medical records for inaccuracies. Upon finding errors, it's their right to submit a written request to the provider's office for an amendment. Whether or not the doctor agrees, the amendment request must be included in the patient's medical record to ensure transparency per the Health Insurance Portability and Accountability Act (HIPAA) Privacy Rule.[1]

14

Before Things Go Sideways

Medical errors can and do derail a patient's life. Filing a complaint with the state medical board, the hospital's administrative office, or a medical malpractice claim may serve little purpose to right a grievous professional wrong. In a just world, it's ethical to report a provider who commits an egregious offense and expect them to be held accountable more often than not. However the unsavory reality is that medical boards consist of volunteer physicians and non-physicians who are inclined to be pro-doctor.[1, 2] What is the point of a medical regulatory board when its members rarely take disciplinary action? As is pervasive throughout the healthcare field, it must be the insatiable desire for social status.

CURIOUS PERSON: "WHAT DO YOU DO?"
BOARD MEMBER: "I SIT ON THE BOARD."
CURIOUS PERSON: "BUT WHAT DO YOU DO?"
BOARD MEMBER: "I JUST TOLD YOU. I SIT. MIND YOU, MERELY SITTING ON THE BOARD IS A FEATHER IN MY CAP."

But as with all feathers, it carries no weight.

When complaints to the state medical board disappear into the healthcare void, aggrieved patients are at liberty to file medical malpractice claims—but winning is a Herculean effort. Horned lawyers make careless doctors look like angels with celestial plumes who do no wrong. Physicians win the majority of medical malpractice claims—even half of all claims where evidence of negligence is strong.[3]

Despite being David and Goliath battles, medical malpractice claims are sometimes won. Regardless, they have little ripple effect: a concerning number of negligent healthcare workers continue to commit gross professional injustices, escape all accountability, and demonstrate zero regard for patient health. The healthcare industry is inundated with practitioners who *do not care*. A number of physicians and nurses do genuinely care and are committed to providing meaningful health*care*. But too many are disguised as healthcare professionals who truly are in the business of for-profit health, viewing vulnerable patients as lucrative income streams.

When professional accountability lacks, there's always...

"YOUR GROSS NEGLIGENCE CAUSED UNNECESSARY PAIN AND SUFFERING TOO? JOIN THE REST OF 'EM. NEXT!"

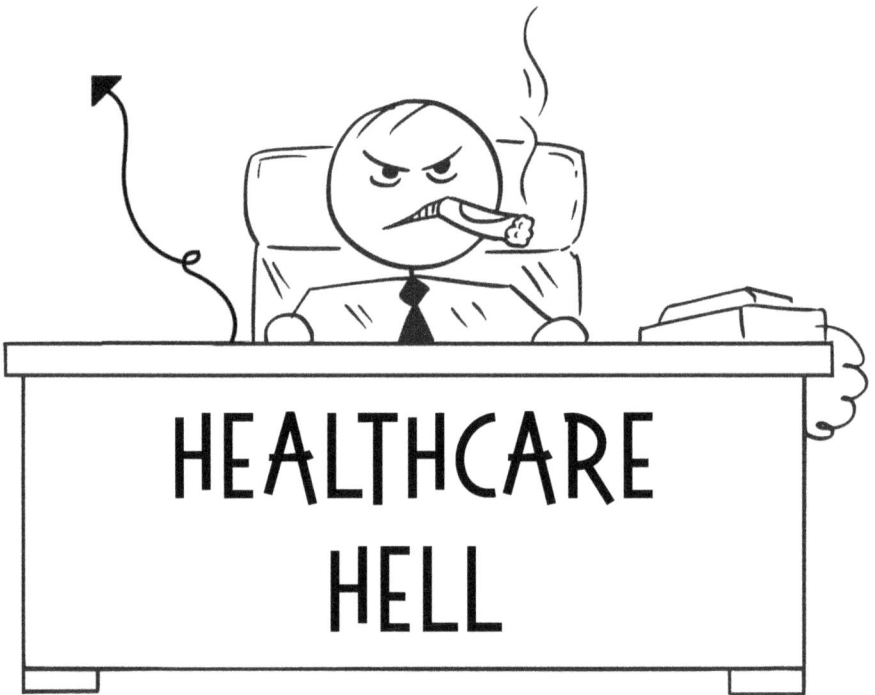

HEALTHCARE HELL

Instead, the wise patient takes steps to *prevent* issues from spiraling into a medical or legal crisis.

Patients who survive the healthcare industry another day...

INVESTIGATE NAGGING SELF-DOUBTS ABOUT A DIAGNOSIS

ASK QUESTIONS—MAKE A LIST, AND CHECK IT TWICE—AND GET ANSWERS

PUT ON THEIR SLEUTH'S HAT AND DO THEIR RESEARCH, RELYING ON MULTIPLE CREDIBLE HEALTH RESOURCES THAT SERVE AS THEIR PERSONAL HEALTH CHAMPIONS

CONSULT ADDITIONAL QUALIFIED HEALTH EXPERTS UNTIL SATISFIED, UNAFRAID OF SEEKING VALIDATING SECOND AND THIRD OPINIONS

LISTEN TO THEIR GUT—UNLESS THEY HAVE GASTROENTERITIS. IN THAT CASE, THEY FIRST CURE THE AWFUL STOMACH FLU, AND THEN TRUST THEIR GUT!

Above all, patients who survive the healthcare industry remain skeptical of recommended health*care*, as it may just as well turn out to be health*abuse*.

15

On Exam the Future Looks Bright

It's a well-known paradox that when doctors go on strike, patient death rates drop or stay the same.[1]

HMM. CAN MEDICAL STRIKES BE BEACONS OF HEALTH?

"DOCTORS ARE ON STRIKE, MADDIE. GUESS I WON'T BE GOING TO THE CLINIC TODAY. I'M NOT FEELING THAT SICK ANYWAY."

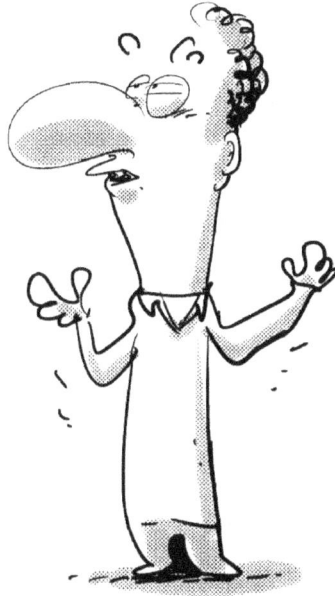

It's not uncommon for healthcare professionals to fail to diagnose disease when worrisome symptoms are present, leaving patients jumping from one doctor to the next, hoping for relief.

It's likewise not unusual for medical experts to translate mild symptoms into serious disease and attempt to convince healthy patients of it too—in these cases, misinformed doctors are like unscrupulous mechanics who tell patients their car needs a pricey, brand-new engine when it's only a loose spark plug that needs a quick tightening.

THE PHYSICIAN SHORTAGE: PROBLEM OR PANACEA?

The US is looming toward a physician shortage. It's a classic case of supply versus demand, spurred by a growing aging population that needs more care coupled with an increasing number of medical doctors ready to hang up the stethoscope in exchange for the sand and sea of retirement.[2]

The anticipated reduction in the doctor workforce presents delightful opportunity for hypothesis:

Does less doctors mean fewer medical mistakes? Does fewer medical mistakes translate to more patient health and well-being? It's a marvel well-worth considering.

SPEAKING OF MEDICAL ERROR...

Artificial intelligence (AI) is metamorphosing society, including the medical community. Some predict AI will outright replace doctors. Others speculate that AI will integrate into medicine in a collaborative manner to enhance patient health outcomes.[3] AI shows superior accuracy in some healthcare aspects but provides overexaggerated results in others—making it quite the mercurial stinker no one wants to rely upon one hundred percent.

Given the promise of AI in enhancing medical accuracy, the future of healthcare seems a tad brighter—but not enough to need shades yet.

For now, and as always, patients rarely benefit from making healthcare decisions out of a lack of knowledge, fear, or naivete. Their body's subtle and not-so-subtle cues are among the most reliable medical advisors that patients could ever consult. Health practitioners are just that—practitioners who respond to those valid advisors with (fingers crossed) skillful action.

SIR STOMACH: "UH, WE'VE GOT TROUBLE RUMBLING."
ADVISEE: "I'M ABOUT TO DOUBLE OVER!"
SIR STOMACH: "YOU BETTER SEE SOMEONE FAST."
HEALTH WORKER: "TAKE TWO OF THESE AND TEXT ME
IN THE MORNING."
SIR STOMACH: "AH, THAT'S BETTER. I'M ALL GOOD."
ADVISEE: "ME TOO."

Is it too late to take charge of your health? As long as you've got a pulse, it's never too late!

Thank You

Thank you for reading *Be Your Best Health Advocate:*
A Journal Empowering Patients to Survive Healthcare Another Day.
If you're not already there, may you be on your way to health!

SALUD!

BONNE SANTE!

L'CHAIM!

SLAINTE!

SALUTE!

GENKI DE NE!

Notes

Chapter 1: The Unhealthy Perception of US Healthcare

1. "Past Deans of the Faculty of Medicine," Harvard Medical School, accessed January 4, 2026, https://hms.harvard.edu/about-hms/office-dean/past-deans-faculty-medicine.

Chapter 2: Charting a New Healthcare Path

1. Jennifer Cole, Chris Watkins, and Dorothea Kleine, "Health Advice From Internet Discussion Forums. How Bad Is Dangerous?," *Journal of Medical Internet Research* 18, no. 1 (January 6, 2016): e4, https://www.jmir.org/2016/1/e4, DOI: 10.2196/jmir.5051.

2. Rachel Feaster, "Do Not Crush List: These Common Medications Should Always Stay Intact," GoodRX, April 4, 2024, https://www.goodrx.com/drugs/medication-basics/do-not-crush-medication-list?srsltid=AfmBOood4q3ZoQGwRQiaXkeVFvjNKmQ0hciT3nlYBlMEQRXAyJgo7uLl.

Chapter 3: Patient (AKA Human) Liberties

1. "Patient Rights | AMA-Code," accessed January 4, 2026, https://code-medical-ethics.ama-assn.org/ethics-opinions/patient-rights.

2. "Patient Bill of Rights and Responsibilities," accessed January 4, 2026, https://www.state.gov/patient-bill-of-rights-and-responsibilities.

Chapter 6: Sizing Up a Diagnosis

1. Nhs Website, "Myalgic Encephalomyelitis or Chronic Fatigue Syndrome (ME/CFS)," nhs.uk, November 11, 2025, https://www.nhs.uk/conditions/chronic-fatigue-syndrome-cfs/#:~:text=There%27s%20no%20specific%20test%20for,have%20blood%20and%20urine%20tests.

2. Carrie MacMillan, "Why More Adults Are Being Diagnosed With Autism," Yale Medicine, September 5, 2025, https://www.yalemedicine.org/news/autism-diagnosis-in-adults.

3. Danielle Lazarowitz, "Why Diagnoses Takes Time (and What You Can Do About It) — Chronius Care," Chronius Care, April 6, 2025, https://www.chronicillnesspcp.com/chronic-thoughts/whats-wrong-with-me-why-getting-diagnosed-can-take-so-long.

4. "The Evolution of Diagnosis: From Ancient Observations to Genetic Insights – HudsonAlpha Institute for Biotechnology," accessed January 18, 2026, https://www.hudsonalpha.org/the-evolution-of-diagnosis-from-ancient-observations-to-genetic-insights/.

Chapter 7: Kicking Off a Medication Regimen

1. "Patient Rights | AMA-Code," accessed January 18, 2026, https://code-medical-ethics.ama-assn.org/ethics-opinions/patient-rights.

Chapter 8: Calling a Medication Quits

1. "Weill Cornell Medical Center | Adverse Effects of Suddenly Stopping a Medicine," accessed January 4, 2026, https://pre.weill.cornell.edu/cert/patients/suddenly_stopping_medicine.html.

2. Center for Drug Evaluation And Research, "Compounding and the FDA: Questions and Answers," U.S. Food And Drug Administration, September 16, 2025, https://www.fda.gov/drugs/human-drug-compounding/compounding-and-fda-questions-and-answers.

Chapter 9: Going Under the Knife

1. Stahel, P.F., VanderHeiden, T.F. & Kim, F.J. "Why do surgeons continue to perform unnecessary surgery?", *Patient Saf Surg* 11, 1 (2017), https://doi.org/10.1186/s13037-016-0117-6.

2. Lo, Yu-Chieh, Yu-Pin Chen, Hui En Lin, Wei-Chun Chang, Wei-Pin Ho, Jia-Pei Jang, and Yi-Jie Kuo. 2025. "Factors Associated with Decisional Regret After Shared Decision Making for Patients Undergoing Total Knee Arthroplasty," *Healthcare* 13, no. 13: 1597. https://doi.org/10.3390/healthcare13131597.

Chapter 10: Less-Squeamish (Non-Surgical) Options

1. Alithea Corter, "Natural Alternatives to Surgery: Exploring Non-Invasive Options," TPC, October 21, 2024, https://tpcportland.com/natural-alternatives-to-surgery/.

Chapter 11: Alt (Alternative) Medicine

1. Erik Enwall, "Alternative Medicine: Pros and Cons," The Southeastern Spine Institute, April 14, 2021, https://southeasternspine.com/alternative-medicine-pros-and-cons/.

2. "Content - Health Encyclopedia - University of Rochester Medical Center," accessed January 18, 2026, https://www.urmc.rochester.edu/encyclopedia/content?contenttypeid=85&contentid=p00171.

3. Matthew Thorpe MD PhD, "How Meditation Benefits Your Mind and Body," Healthline, August 15, 2024, https://www.healthline.com/nutrition/12-benefits-of-meditation#accessibility.

4. Caballero-Gallardo, Karina, Patricia Quintero-Rincón, and Jesus Olivero-Verbel. 2025. "Aromatherapy and Essential Oils: Holistic Strategies in Complementary and Alternative Medicine for Integral Wellbeing," *Plants* 14, no. 3: 400. https://doi.org/10.3390/plants14030400.

5. Anton C. De Groot and Erich Schmidt, "Essential Oils, Part IV: Contact Allergy," *Dermatitis: contact, atopic, occupational, drug* 27, no. 4 (July 1, 2016): 170–75, doi:10.1097/DER.0000000000000197, https://pubmed.ncbi.nlm.nih.gov/27427818/.

6. "How Do I Determine the Quality of Essential Oils?," Taking Charge of Your Wellbeing, December 31, 1969, https://www.takingcharge.csh.umn.edu/how-do-i-determine-quality-essential-oils.

7. Qing Li, "Effects of Forest Environment (Shinrin-yoku/Forest Bathing) on Health Promotion and Disease Prevention — the Establishment of 'Forest Medicine'—," *Environmental Health and Preventive Medicine* 27, no. 0 (January 1, 2022): 43, https://doi.org/10.1265/ehpm.22-00160.

8. Physiopedia contributors, "Sunlight, Outdoor Light, and Light Therapy in Disease Management," *Physiopedia*, accessed January 18, 2026, https://www.physio-pedia.com/index.php?title=Sunlight,_Outdoor_Light,_and_Light_Therapy_in_Disease_Management&oldid=290319

Chapter 12: Lifestyle Upgrades

1. Gabbi Shaw and Kim Schewitz, "10 Celebrities Who Lived to 100 — and How They Did It," Business Insider, September 25, 2025, https://www.businessinsider.com/celebrities-who-lived-to-100-longevity-tips-george-burns-9.

2. "The Water in You: Water and the Human Body," USGS, October 22, 2019, https://www.usgs.gov/water-science-school/science/water-you-water-and-human-body.

3. National Library of Medicine, "Dehydration," accessed January 18, 2026, https://medlineplus.gov/dehydration.html.

4. Wayne Gao, PhD, Mattia Sanna, PhD, and Yea-Hung Chen, PhD, "Occupational Sitting Time, Leisure Physical Activity, and All-Cause and Cardiovascular Disease Mortality," JAMA Network, January 19, 2024, https://jamanetwork.com/journals/jamanetworkopen/fullarticle/2814094#249495009.

5. "Adult Activity: An Overview," Physical Activity Basics, December 20, 2023, https://www.cdc.gov/physical-activity-basics/guidelines/adults.html.

6. "Health Effects of Social Isolation and Loneliness," Social Connection, May 15, 2024, https://www.cdc.gov/social-connectedness/risk-factors/index.html.

7. "Improve Your Emotional Well-Being," Emotional Well-Being, August 26, 2024, https://www.cdc.gov/emotional-well-being/improve-your-emotional-well-being/index.html.

8. eClinicalMedicine, "Letting Happiness Happen," *EClinicalMedicine* 86 (August 1, 2025): 103467, https://doi.org/10.1016/j.eclinm.2025.103467.

Chapter 13: The Boring-But-Necessary Medical Records Review

1. "45 CFR 164.526 -- Amendment of Protected Health Information.," accessed January 4, 2026, https://www.ecfr.gov/current/title-45/subtitle-A/subchapter-C/part-164/subpart-E/section-164.526.

Chapter 14: Before Things Go Sideways

1. "US Medical Regulatory Trends and Actions," Federation of State Medical Boards, accessed January 4, 2026, https://www.fsmb.org/u.s.-medical-regulatory-trends-and-actions/guide-to-medical-

regulation-in-the-united-states/introduction/

2. Gina Barton, Ahcj Staff, "Records Show 'Dangerous Doctors' Rarely Face Discipline," Association of Health Care Journalists, October 9, 2023, https://healthjournalism.org/blog/2008/06/records-show-dangerous-doctors-rarely-face-discipline/.

3. Philip G. Peters Jr., "Doctors & Juries," 105 MICH. L. REV. 1453 (2007), accessed January 19, 2026, https://repository.law.umich.edu/mlr/vol105/iss7/7

Chapter 15: On Exam the Future Looks Bright

1. Daniel Avdic et al., "Alive and Kicking? Short-Term Health Effects of a Physician Strike in Germany," CMEPR, September 27, 2023, https://cmepr.gmu.edu/wp-content/uploads/2023/09/Avdic-et-al.pdf.

2. Abdel-Razig, Sawsan, and James K Stoller. "Addressing Physician Shortages in the United States With Novel Legislation to Bypass Traditional Training Pathways: The Fine Print." *Journal of Graduate Medical Education* vol. 17,1: 16-19, February 4, 2025, https://jgme.kglmeridian.com/view/journals/jgme/17/1/article-p16.xml?body=FullText

3. Jennifer Grebow, "Can Artificial Intelligence Replace Doctors?," Keck Medicine of USC, April 23, 2025, https://www.keckmedicine.org/physician-hub/can-artificial-intelligence-replace-doctors/.

.